THE IBS COOKBOOK FOR SENIORS

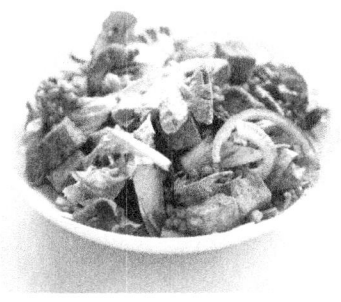

DR. JESSICA SMITH

Copyright © 2024 by DR. JESSICA SMITH

All rights reserved.

No part of this book may be reproduced, stored in a retrieval system, or transmitted, in any form or by any means, electronic, mechanical, photocopying, recording, or otherwise, without prior written permission from the publisher, except for brief quotations embodied in critical articles or reviews.

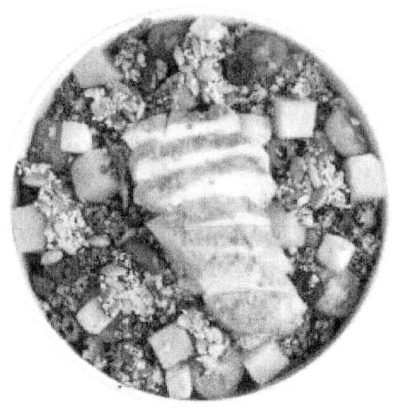

TABLE OF CONTENTS

CHAPTER ONE 7

How to Use this Cookbook 7

Understanding Ibs Recipes for Seniors 9

Benefits of Ibs Recipes for Seniors 11

Guidelines for Ibs Recipes for Seniors 13

Causes of Ibs in Seniors 15

Symptoms of Ibs in Seniors 17

Risk Factor of Ibs in Seniors 19

CHAPTER TWO 21

IBS Breakfast Recipes for Seniors 21

1: Low-FODMAP Banana Oatmeal 21

2: Scrambled Tofu with Spinach 22

3: Blueberry Almond Smoothie Bowl 24

4: Quinoa Breakfast Porridge 25

5: Chia Seed Pudding with Mixed Berries 27

6: Spinach and Tomato Frittata 28

7: Rice Cake with Peanut Butter and Banana ... 30

8: Yogurt Parfait with Granola and Berries 31

9: Veggie Omelette 32

10: Overnight Chia Seed Pudding 34

IBS Lunch Recipes for Seniors 35

1: Quinoa Salad with Chicken and Vegetables 35

2: Turkey and Avocado Wrap 37

3: Salmon and Quinoa Salad 39

4: Turkey and Quinoa Stuffed Bell Peppers 41

5: Tuna Salad Lettuce Wraps 43

6: Quinoa and Vegetable Stir-Fry 44

7: Quinoa and Chicken Soup 47

8: Shrimp and Avocado Salad 48

9: Lentil and Vegetable Soup 50

10: Turkey and Vegetable Stir-Fry 52

IBS Dinner Recipes for Seniors 54

1: Lemon Herb Baked Salmon with Quinoa and Steamed Vegetables 54

2: Turkey and Vegetable Stir-Fry with Brown Rice 56

3: Baked Chicken Breast with Roasted Vegetables 58

4: Quinoa and Black Bean Stuffed Bell Peppers 60

5: Turkey and Vegetable Soup 62

6: Baked Cod with Lemon and Herbs 64

7: Grilled Chicken and Vegetable Skewers 66

8: Turkey and Quinoa Stuffed Bell Peppers 68

9: Salmon and Vegetable Foil Packets 70

10: Turkey and Vegetable Quinoa Bowl 72

IBS Snacks Recipes for Seniors 74

1: Rice Cake with Avocado and Tomato 74

2: Greek Yogurt with Berries and Almonds 76

3: Carrot Sticks with Hummus 77

4: Rice Cake with Almond Butter and Banana. 78

5: Quinoa Salad with Cucumber and Feta 79

6: Rice Crackers with Tuna Salad 81

7: Baked Sweet Potato Chips 82

8: Cottage Cheese with Pineapple 84

9: Almond Butter and Banana Roll-Ups 85

10: Veggie Sticks with Yogurt Dip 87

CONCLUSION 89

CHAPTER ONE

How to Use this Cookbook

Understanding IBS

Begin by familiarizing yourself with Irritable Bowel Syndrome (IBS), its symptoms, triggers, and how it affects digestion. This knowledge will help you make informed choices when selecting recipes.

Consultation with a Healthcare Professional

Before making any significant changes to your diet, consult with a healthcare professional, preferably a nutritionist or dietitian. They can offer personalized advice tailored to your specific needs and health conditions.

Identifying Trigger Foods

Work with your healthcare professional to identify trigger foods that exacerbate your IBS symptoms. Common triggers include dairy, gluten, certain vegetables, and spicy foods. Knowing your triggers will help you select suitable recipes.

Stocking Up on IBS-Friendly Ingredients Create a list of IBS-friendly ingredients such as low-FODMAP fruits and vegetables, lean proteins, gluten-free grains, and lactose-free dairy alternatives. Stock up on these ingredients to have them readily available when preparing recipes.

Selecting Recipes

Choose recipes from "**The IBS Recipes Cookbook for Seniors**" that align with your dietary restrictions and preferences. Look for recipes that use low-FODMAP ingredients and are gentle on the digestive system.

Meal Planning

Plan your meals in advance to ensure a balanced and varied diet. Aim for a combination of protein, carbohydrates, healthy fats, and fiber in each meal. Incorporate recipes from the cookbook into your meal plan for a diverse range of flavors and nutrients.

Cooking Techniques

Experiment with different cooking techniques such as steaming, baking, grilling, and sautéing to prepare delicious and easy-to-digest meals. Avoid deep-frying or heavily processed foods, as they can aggravate IBS symptoms.

Portion Control: Practice portion control to prevent overeating, which can lead to discomfort and worsen IBS symptoms. Use smaller plates and bowls to help manage portion sizes and listen to your body's hunger and fullness cues.

Hydration

Stay hydrated by drinking plenty of water throughout the day. Limit intake of caffeinated and carbonated beverages, as they can irritate the digestive system. Opt for herbal teas or infused water as refreshing alternatives.

Enjoying Meals Mindfully

Take your time to savor each meal, chewing slowly and mindfully. Pay attention to how different foods make you feel and adjust your diet accordingly. Enjoying meals in a relaxed environment can help alleviate stress and improve digestion.

Understanding Ibs Recipes for Seniors

Understanding IBS (Irritable Bowel Syndrome) and its impact on seniors is crucial for creating effective recipes tailored to their needs.

IBS is a common gastrointestinal disorder characterized by symptoms such as abdominal pain, bloating, gas, diarrhea, and constipation. For seniors, managing IBS becomes even more critical as age-related changes in digestion may exacerbate symptoms.

IBS recipes for seniors focus on incorporating ingredients that are gentle on the digestive system while providing essential nutrients.

These recipes often adhere to the low-FODMAP diet, which restricts fermentable carbohydrates that can trigger IBS symptoms.

Seniors with IBS may find relief by avoiding certain foods such as dairy, gluten, high-fat foods, caffeine, and spicy foods.

When crafting IBS recipes for seniors, it's essential to prioritize easily digestible ingredients such as lean proteins, low-FODMAP fruits and vegetables, gluten-free grains, and lactose-free dairy alternatives.

Cooking techniques that promote digestibility, such as steaming, baking, and grilling, are preferred over frying or heavy processing.

Moreover, portion control and mindful eating play significant roles in managing IBS symptoms. Seniors should be encouraged to eat smaller, frequent meals and chew food slowly to aid digestion.

Hydration is also essential, as adequate water intake helps maintain bowel regularity and prevent dehydration, which can exacerbate symptoms.

In essence, understanding IBS and tailoring recipes to seniors' needs can significantly improve their quality of life by reducing symptoms and promoting overall digestive health.

Benefits of Ibs Recipes for Seniors

IBS recipes tailored for seniors offer a multitude of benefits that contribute to their overall well-being and quality of life.

Here are some key advantages:

Symptom Management: IBS recipes focus on ingredients that are gentle on the digestive system, helping seniors manage uncomfortable symptoms such as abdominal pain, bloating, gas, diarrhea, and constipation.

By avoiding trigger foods and following dietary guidelines, seniors can experience reduced frequency and severity of IBS flare-ups.

Improved Nutritional Intake: Seniors with IBS may struggle to obtain adequate nutrition due to dietary restrictions and digestive issues. IBS recipes prioritize nutrient-dense ingredients, ensuring seniors receive essential vitamins, minerals, and antioxidants necessary for optimal health. By incorporating a variety of whole foods into their diet, seniors can maintain better overall nutrition.

Enhanced Digestive Health: The emphasis on easily digestible ingredients and cooking techniques in IBS recipes promotes better digestion and gut health for seniors. By choosing foods that are less likely to cause irritation or inflammation in the digestive tract, seniors can experience improved bowel regularity and reduced discomfort.

Increased Energy and Vitality: By providing seniors with balanced, nourishing meals, IBS recipes can boost energy levels and vitality. Proper nutrition supports overall physical health and mental well-being, allowing seniors to engage in daily activities with greater ease and enjoyment.

Quality of Life Improvement: Ultimately, IBS recipes contribute to a better quality of life for seniors by helping them manage their condition effectively, enjoy delicious and satisfying meals, and maintain their independence and dignity in their golden years.

Guidelines for Ibs Recipes for Seniors

Crafting IBS recipes specifically tailored for seniors involves adhering to certain guidelines to ensure the meals are both nutritious and gentle on the digestive system.

Here are some essential guidelines:

Low-FODMAP Ingredients: Focus on incorporating low-FODMAP foods into recipes. These include easily digestible fruits and vegetables such as berries, bananas, carrots, and spinach, as well as lean proteins like chicken, fish, and tofu. Limit high-FODMAP foods such as onions, garlic, and certain legumes, which can exacerbate IBS symptoms.

Fiber-Rich Foods: Choose fiber-rich ingredients such as oats, quinoa, and brown rice, which support digestive health and help alleviate constipation. However, be mindful of insoluble fiber, which may aggravate symptoms in some individuals. Gradually increase fiber intake to avoid discomfort.

Healthy Fats: Opt for sources of healthy fats such as avocado, nuts, seeds, and olive oil. These fats provide essential nutrients and promote satiety without exacerbating digestive issues.

Limit Trigger Foods: Identify trigger foods that exacerbate IBS symptoms and avoid or minimize their use in recipes. Common triggers include dairy, gluten, spicy foods, caffeine, and alcohol. Replace these ingredients with suitable alternatives to prevent discomfort.

Cooking Techniques: Use gentle cooking techniques such as steaming, baking, and grilling to prepare meals. Avoid frying or heavy processing, which can make foods harder to digest and worsen symptoms.

Portion Control: Practice portion control to prevent overeating, which can lead to discomfort and exacerbate IBS symptoms. Serve smaller, more frequent meals throughout the day to support digestion.

Hydration: Encourage seniors to stay hydrated by drinking plenty of water throughout the day. Limit intake of caffeinated and carbonated beverages, as they can irritate the digestive system.

Monitor and Adjust: Pay attention to how seniors respond to different ingredients and recipes. Monitor their symptoms and adjust recipes accordingly to better suit their individual needs and preferences. Regularly consult with healthcare professionals for personalized guidance and support.

Causes of Ibs in Seniors

Irritable Bowel Syndrome (IBS) in seniors can be attributed to various factors, including physiological changes, lifestyle factors, and underlying health conditions.

Here are some common causes of IBS in seniors:

Aging Digestive System: As individuals age, the digestive system undergoes natural changes, such as decreased gastrointestinal motility and reduced production of digestive enzymes. These age-related changes can contribute to symptoms of IBS, including altered bowel habits and increased sensitivity to certain foods.

Diet: Poor dietary habits, such as consuming large amounts of fatty or spicy foods, inadequate fiber intake, and irregular meal patterns, can trigger or exacerbate IBS symptoms in seniors. Certain foods and beverages, such as dairy products, caffeine, alcohol, and artificial sweeteners, may also worsen symptoms.

Stress: Stress can have a significant impact on digestive health and may exacerbate symptoms of IBS in seniors. Life transitions, emotional stressors, and changes in routine associated with aging can all contribute to heightened stress levels, potentially triggering IBS flare-ups.

Medications: Seniors often take multiple medications to manage various health conditions, some of which may have gastrointestinal side effects or disrupt the balance of gut bacteria, contributing to IBS symptoms.

Underlying Health Conditions: Seniors may have underlying health conditions, such as diverticulosis, gastrointestinal infections, or inflammatory bowel disease (IBD), that can mimic or exacerbate symptoms of IBS. Identifying and managing these conditions is essential for effectively addressing IBS symptoms in seniors.

Hormonal Changes: Fluctuations in hormone levels, particularly in post-menopausal women, may influence digestive function and contribute to the development or worsening of IBS symptoms.

Understanding the causes of IBS in seniors is crucial for implementing effective management strategies and improving their quality of life.

A comprehensive approach that addresses diet, stress management, medication management, and underlying health conditions is key to managing IBS effectively in this population.

Symptoms of Ibs in Seniors

Symptoms of Irritable Bowel Syndrome (IBS) in seniors can vary widely in both presentation and severity. While some seniors may experience mild discomfort, others may have more debilitating symptoms that significantly impact their quality of life.

Here are common symptoms of IBS in seniors:

Abdominal Pain and Cramping: Seniors with IBS often experience abdominal discomfort or cramping, which may range from mild to severe and can occur intermittently or persistently.

Altered Bowel Habits: IBS can cause changes in bowel habits, including diarrhea, constipation, or alternating between the two. Seniors may experience urgency or difficulty with bowel movements, leading to frustration and discomfort.

Bloating and Gas: Many seniors with IBS experience bloating, a sensation of fullness, and excessive gas, which can contribute to abdominal discomfort and social embarrassment.

Fatigue: Chronic symptoms of IBS, such as pain, disrupted sleep, and psychological distress, can lead to fatigue and decreased energy levels in seniors.

Nausea and Indigestion: Some seniors with IBS may experience symptoms of nausea, indigestion, and acid reflux, which can further contribute to discomfort and disrupt daily activities.

Psychological Symptoms: IBS is often associated with psychological symptoms such as anxiety, depression, and stress, which can exacerbate gastrointestinal symptoms and impair quality of life in seniors.

Other Symptoms: Additional symptoms of IBS in seniors may include mucus in the stool, incomplete bowel movements, and urinary symptoms such as urgency or frequency.

It's important for seniors experiencing these symptoms to consult with a healthcare professional for proper diagnosis and management of IBS.

Treatment may involve lifestyle modifications, dietary changes, medication, and stress management techniques to alleviate symptoms and improve overall well-being.

Risk Factor of Ibs in Seniors

Seniors may face specific risk factors that predispose them to developing Irritable Bowel Syndrome (IBS) or exacerbate existing symptoms. Understanding these risk factors is crucial for effective management and prevention.

Here are some key risk factors for IBS in seniors:

Age-related Changes: As individuals age, the digestive system undergoes natural changes, including decreased gastrointestinal motility and reduced production of digestive enzymes. These age-related changes can increase the risk of developing IBS or worsen existing symptoms in seniors.

Dietary Habits: Poor dietary habits, such as consuming high-fat or spicy foods, inadequate fiber intake, and irregular meal patterns, can contribute to the development or exacerbation of IBS symptoms in seniors. Certain foods and beverages, such as dairy products, caffeine, alcohol, and artificial sweeteners, may also trigger symptoms.

Stress and Anxiety: Seniors may experience significant life stressors, such as retirement, loss of loved ones, or health concerns, which can contribute to heightened stress and anxiety levels.

Medications: Seniors often take multiple medications to manage various health conditions, some of which may have gastrointestinal side effects or disrupt the balance of gut bacteria, increasing the risk of developing or worsening IBS symptoms.

Hormonal Changes: Fluctuations in hormone levels, particularly in post-menopausal women, may influence digestive function and contribute to the development or worsening of IBS symptoms in seniors

CHAPTER TWO

IBS Breakfast Recipes for Seniors

1: Low-FODMAP Banana Oatmeal

Ingredients:

- 1 ripe banana, mashed
- 1/2 cup gluten-free rolled oats
- 1 cup lactose-free milk or almond milk
- 1 tablespoon maple syrup (optional)
- 1 tablespoon chia seeds (optional)
- 1/4 teaspoon ground cinnamon
- Toppings: sliced strawberries, blueberries, or raspberries (low-FODMAP fruits)

Instructions:

- In a small saucepan, combine mashed banana, rolled oats, lactose-free milk, maple syrup (if using), chia seeds (if using), and ground cinnamon.
- Bring the mixture to a gentle boil over medium heat, stirring occasionally.

- Reduce heat to low and simmer for 5-7 minutes, or until the oats are cooked and the mixture thickens to your desired consistency.
- Remove from heat and let it sit for a minute to cool slightly.
- Serve warm topped with sliced low-FODMAP fruits like strawberries, blueberries, or raspberries.

Health Benefits:

- Bananas provide potassium and fiber, which support heart health and digestive regularity.
- Oats are a good source of soluble fiber, which helps stabilize blood sugar levels and promote satiety.
- Chia seeds are rich in omega-3 fatty acids and fiber, which support heart health and digestive function.

Preparation Time: 10 minutes

2: Scrambled Tofu with Spinach

Ingredients:

- 1/2 block extra-firm tofu, crumbled
- 1 cup fresh spinach, chopped
- 1 tablespoon olive oil

- 1/4 teaspoon turmeric powder
- Salt and pepper to taste

Instructions:

- Heat olive oil in a skillet over medium heat.
- Add crumbled tofu to the skillet and cook for 3-4 minutes, stirring occasionally.
- Add chopped spinach to the skillet and continue to cook for another 2-3 minutes, or until the spinach wilts and the tofu is heated through.
- Sprinkle turmeric powder over the tofu and spinach mixture, stirring to combine. Season with salt and pepper to taste.
- Remove from heat and serve hot.

Health Benefits:

- Tofu is a plant-based source of protein and contains essential amino acids necessary for muscle health and repair.
- Spinach is rich in vitamins A, C, and K, as well as folate and iron, which support immune function and blood health.

Preparation Time: 15 minutes

3: Blueberry Almond Smoothie Bowl

Ingredients:

- 1 ripe banana, frozen
- 1/2 cup frozen blueberries
- 1/4 cup almond butter
- 1/2 cup lactose-free yogurt or almond milk
- 1 tablespoon chia seeds
- Toppings: sliced almonds, shredded coconut, fresh blueberries

Instructions:

- In a blender, combine the frozen banana, frozen blueberries, almond butter, lactose-free yogurt or almond milk, and chia seeds.
- Blend until smooth and creamy, adding more liquid if necessary to achieve your desired consistency.
- Pour the smoothie into a bowl and top with sliced almonds, shredded coconut, and fresh blueberries.
- Serve immediately and enjoy with a spoon.

Health Benefits:

- Blueberries are rich in antioxidants and fiber, which support heart health and digestive regularity.
- Almond butter provides healthy fats, protein, and vitamin E, which promote satiety and overall well-being.
- Chia seeds are a good source of omega-3 fatty acids and fiber, which support heart health and digestive function.

Preparation Time: 5 minutes

4: Quinoa Breakfast Porridge

Ingredients:

- 1/2 cup quinoa, rinsed
- 1 cup water or lactose-free milk
- 1/2 teaspoon ground cinnamon
- 1/4 teaspoon vanilla extract
- 1 tablespoon maple syrup (optional)
- Toppings: sliced bananas, chopped walnuts, drizzle of honey (optional)

Instructions:

- In a small saucepan, combine quinoa, water or lactose-free milk, ground cinnamon, and vanilla extract.
- Bring the mixture to a boil over medium heat, then reduce heat to low and simmer for 15-20 minutes, or until the quinoa is cooked and the mixture thickens.
- Stir in maple syrup (if using) and continue to cook for another minute.
- Remove from heat and let it sit for a minute to cool slightly.
- Serve warm topped with sliced bananas, chopped walnuts, and a drizzle of honey (if using).

Health Benefits:

- Quinoa is a gluten-free whole grain that provides protein, fiber, and essential nutrients, supporting overall health and digestion.
- Cinnamon has anti-inflammatory properties and may help regulate blood sugar levels, promoting stable energy levels throughout the day.

Preparation Time: 25 minutes

5: Chia Seed Pudding with Mixed Berries

Ingredients:

- 2 tablespoons chia seeds
- 1/2 cup lactose-free milk or almond milk
- 1/4 teaspoon vanilla extract
- 1 tablespoon maple syrup (optional)
- Mixed berries (e.g., strawberries, raspberries, blueberries) for topping

Instructions:

- In a bowl, mix chia seeds, lactose-free milk or almond milk, vanilla extract, and maple syrup (if using).
- Stir well to combine, ensuring that the chia seeds are evenly distributed.
- Cover the bowl and refrigerate for at least 2 hours or overnight, allowing the chia seeds to absorb the liquid and form a pudding-like consistency.
- Once the chia seed pudding has set, remove it from the refrigerator and give it a good stir.
- Serve the pudding in individual bowls and top with mixed berries.

- Enjoy cold for a refreshing and nutritious breakfast.

Health Benefits:

- Chia seeds are rich in omega-3 fatty acids, fiber, and antioxidants, promoting heart health and digestive regularity.
- Berries are packed with vitamins, minerals, and phytonutrients, supporting immune function and overall well-being.

Preparation Time: 5 minutes (plus chilling time)

6: Spinach and Tomato Frittata

Ingredients:

- 4 large eggs
- 1 cup fresh spinach, chopped
- 1/2 cup cherry tomatoes, halved
- 1/4 cup lactose-free milk or almond milk
- Salt and pepper to taste
- 1 tablespoon olive oil

Instructions:

- Preheat the oven to 350°F (175°C).

- In a bowl, whisk together eggs, lactose-free milk or almond milk, salt, and pepper until well combined.
- Heat olive oil in an oven-safe skillet over medium heat.
- Add chopped spinach and cherry tomatoes to the skillet, cooking until the spinach wilts and the tomatoes soften slightly.
- Pour the egg mixture over the spinach and tomatoes, ensuring that the ingredients are evenly distributed.
- Cook for 3-4 minutes, or until the edges of the frittata begin to set.
- Transfer the skillet to the preheated oven and bake for 10-12 minutes, or until the frittata is cooked through and set in the center.
- Remove from the oven and let it cool slightly before slicing into wedges.
- Serve warm and enjoy as a hearty breakfast option.

Health Benefits:

- Eggs provide high-quality protein and essential nutrients, supporting muscle health and overall well-being.

- Spinach and tomatoes are rich in vitamins, minerals, and antioxidants, promoting immune function and cardiovascular health.

Preparation Time: 20 minutes

7: Rice Cake with Peanut Butter and Banana

Ingredients:

- 1 rice cake (gluten-free if necessary)
- 1 tablespoon natural peanut butter (or almond butter for variety)
- 1/2 ripe banana, thinly sliced
- 1 teaspoon honey (optional)
- Pinch of cinnamon (optional)

Instructions:

- Spread the peanut butter evenly over the rice cake.
- Top with thinly sliced banana.
- Drizzle with honey and sprinkle with cinnamon if desired.
- Serve immediately and enjoy as a quick and easy breakfast option.

Health Benefits:

- Rice cakes provide a gluten-free, low-FODMAP base for the breakfast option.
- Peanut butter offers healthy fats and protein, providing energy and satiety.
- Bananas are a good source of potassium and fiber, promoting digestive health and heart health.

Preparation Time: 5 minutes

8: Yogurt Parfait with Granola and Berries

Ingredients:

- 1/2 cup lactose-free yogurt or Greek yogurt
- 1/4 cup low-FODMAP granola (gluten-free if necessary)
- 1/4 cup mixed berries (e.g., strawberries, blueberries, raspberries)

Instructions:

- In a glass or bowl, layer lactose-free yogurt, granola, and mixed berries.
- Repeat the layers until all ingredients are used, ending with a layer of berries on top.

- Serve immediately and enjoy as a refreshing and satisfying breakfast option.

Health Benefits:

- Yogurt provides probiotics and protein, supporting gut health and muscle health.
- Low-FODMAP granola offers fiber and complex carbohydrates, providing sustained energy and digestive regularity.
- Berries are rich in antioxidants and vitamins, promoting immune function and overall well-being.

Preparation Time: 5 minutes

9: Veggie Omelette

Ingredients:

- 2 large eggs
- 1/4 cup chopped bell peppers (red, green, or yellow)
- 1/4 cup chopped zucchini
- 1/4 cup chopped tomatoes
- 1 tablespoon chopped fresh parsley
- Salt and pepper to taste
- 1 teaspoon olive oil

Instructions:

- In a bowl, beat the eggs until well combined. Stir in chopped bell peppers, zucchini, tomatoes, and parsley. Season with salt and pepper.
- Heat olive oil in a non-stick skillet over medium heat.
- Pour the egg mixture into the skillet, spreading it out evenly.
- Cook for 2-3 minutes, or until the edges begin to set.
- Using a spatula, gently lift the edges of the omelette and tilt the skillet to allow any uncooked egg to flow to the bottom.
- Continue cooking for another 2-3 minutes, or until the omelette is cooked through and golden brown on the bottom.
- Carefully fold the omelette in half using the spatula.
- Slide the omelette onto a plate and serve hot.

Health Benefits:

- Eggs provide high-quality protein and essential nutrients, supporting muscle health and overall well-being.

- Bell peppers, zucchini, and tomatoes are rich in vitamins, minerals, and antioxidants, promoting immune function and heart health.

Preparation Time: 10 minutes

10: Overnight Chia Seed Pudding

Ingredients:

- 2 tablespoons chia seeds
- 1/2 cup lactose-free milk or almond milk
- 1/4 teaspoon vanilla extract
- 1 tablespoon maple syrup or honey (optional)
- Sliced fruit for topping (e.g., strawberries, kiwi, mango)

Instructions:

- In a jar or bowl, mix chia seeds, lactose-free milk or almond milk, vanilla extract, and maple syrup or honey (if using).
- Stir well to combine, ensuring that the chia seeds are evenly distributed.

- Cover the jar or bowl and refrigerate overnight, allowing the chia seeds to absorb the liquid and form a pudding-like consistency.
- Once the chia seed pudding has set, remove it from the refrigerator and give it a good stir.
- Top with sliced fruit before serving.
- Enjoy cold as a refreshing and nutritious breakfast option.

Health Benefits:

- Chia seeds are rich in omega-3 fatty acids, fiber, and antioxidants, promoting heart health and digestive regularity.
- Lactose-free milk or almond milk provides calcium and vitamin D, supporting bone health and immune function.

Preparation Time: 5 minutes (plus chilling time)

IBS Lunch Recipes for Seniors

1: Quinoa Salad with Chicken and Vegetables

Ingredients:

- 1/2 cup quinoa, rinsed

- 1 cup water
- 1 boneless, skinless chicken breast, cooked and shredded
- 1 cup mixed vegetables (e.g., bell peppers, cucumber, cherry tomatoes)
- 2 tablespoons chopped fresh parsley
- 2 tablespoons olive oil
- 1 tablespoon lemon juice
- Salt and pepper to taste

Instructions:

- In a saucepan, combine quinoa and water. Bring to a boil, then reduce heat to low and simmer, covered, for 15 minutes or until quinoa is cooked and water is absorbed. Remove from heat and let it cool.
- In a large bowl, combine cooked quinoa, shredded chicken, mixed vegetables, and chopped parsley.
- In a small bowl, whisk together olive oil, lemon juice, salt, and pepper to make the dressing.
- Pour the dressing over the quinoa salad and toss gently to combine.

- Serve immediately or refrigerate for later. Enjoy cold or at room temperature.

Health Benefits:

- Quinoa is a gluten-free whole grain rich in protein and fiber, promoting digestive health and providing sustained energy.
- Chicken is a lean source of protein, essential for muscle health and repair.
- Mixed vegetables provide vitamins, minerals, and antioxidants, supporting immune function and overall well-being.

Preparation Time: 25 minutes

2: Turkey and Avocado Wrap

Ingredients:

- 1 gluten-free tortilla wrap
- 2 ounces cooked turkey breast, sliced
- 1/4 avocado, sliced
- 1/4 cup shredded lettuce
- 1/4 cup sliced cucumber
- 1 tablespoon hummus (optional)

- Salt and pepper to taste

Instructions:

- Lay the tortilla wrap flat on a clean surface.
- Spread hummus (if using) evenly over the tortilla.
- Layer sliced turkey breast, avocado, shredded lettuce, and sliced cucumber on top of the tortilla.
- Season with salt and pepper to taste.
- Roll up the tortilla tightly, tucking in the sides as you go.
- Slice the wrap in half diagonally.
- Serve immediately or wrap in foil for later. Enjoy as a convenient and satisfying lunch option.

Health Benefits:

- Turkey is a lean source of protein and provides essential amino acids necessary for muscle health and repair.
- Avocado is rich in heart-healthy monounsaturated fats and fiber, promoting satiety and supporting digestive health.

- Gluten-free tortilla wraps offer a convenient and easily digestible alternative for individuals with IBS and gluten sensitivities.

Preparation Time: 10 minutes

3: Salmon and Quinoa Salad

Ingredients:

- 1/2 cup quinoa, rinsed
- 1 cup water
- 4 ounces cooked salmon, flaked
- 1 cup mixed greens (e.g., spinach, arugula, kale)
- 1/4 cup cherry tomatoes, halved
- 1/4 cup sliced cucumber
- 2 tablespoons chopped fresh dill
- 2 tablespoons olive oil
- 1 tablespoon lemon juice
- Salt and pepper to taste

Instructions:

- In a saucepan, combine quinoa and water. Bring to a boil, then reduce heat to low and simmer, covered,

for 15 minutes or until quinoa is cooked and water is absorbed. Remove from heat and let it cool.
- In a large bowl, combine cooked quinoa, flaked salmon, mixed greens, cherry tomatoes, sliced cucumber, and chopped dill.
- In a small bowl, whisk together olive oil, lemon juice, salt, and pepper to make the dressing.
- Pour the dressing over the salad and toss gently to combine.
- Serve immediately or refrigerate for later. Enjoy cold or at room temperature.

Health Benefits:

- Salmon is rich in omega-3 fatty acids, protein, and vitamin D, promoting heart health and supporting brain function.
- Quinoa is a gluten-free whole grain rich in protein, fiber, and essential nutrients, providing sustained energy and promoting digestive health.
- Mixed greens, cherry tomatoes, and cucumber provide vitamins, minerals, and antioxidants, supporting immune function and overall well-being.

Preparation Time: 25 minutes

4: Turkey and Quinoa Stuffed Bell Peppers

Ingredients:

- 2 large bell peppers, halved and seeds removed
- 1/2 cup quinoa, rinsed
- 1 cup water
- 4 ounces cooked turkey breast, diced
- 1/4 cup diced tomatoes
- 1/4 cup diced zucchini
- 1/4 cup diced carrots
- 2 tablespoons chopped fresh parsley
- 1 tablespoon olive oil
- 1/2 teaspoon garlic powder
- Salt and pepper to taste

Instructions:

- Preheat the oven to 375°F (190°C). Place the halved bell peppers in a baking dish, cut side up.
- In a saucepan, combine quinoa and water. Bring to a boil, then reduce heat to low and simmer, covered,

for 15 minutes or until quinoa is cooked and water is absorbed. Remove from heat and let it cool.

- In a large bowl, combine cooked quinoa, diced turkey breast, diced tomatoes, diced zucchini, diced carrots, chopped parsley, olive oil, garlic powder, salt, and pepper.
- Spoon the quinoa mixture evenly into the halved bell peppers.
- Cover the baking dish with aluminum foil and bake in the preheated oven for 25-30 minutes, or until the bell peppers are tender.
- Remove from the oven and let them cool slightly before serving.

Health Benefits:

- Bell peppers are rich in vitamins A and C, antioxidants, and fiber, promoting eye health and immune function.
- Turkey provides lean protein, essential amino acids, and vitamin B6, supporting muscle health and overall well-being.

- Quinoa is a gluten-free whole grain rich in protein, fiber, and essential nutrients, providing sustained energy and promoting digestive health.

Preparation Time: 40 minutes

5: Tuna Salad Lettuce Wraps

Ingredients:

- 1 can (5 ounces) tuna, drained
- 2 tablespoons mayonnaise (or dairy-free alternative)
- 1 tablespoon Dijon mustard
- 1 tablespoon lemon juice
- 1/4 cup finely chopped celery
- 1/4 cup finely chopped red onion (optional)
- Salt and pepper to taste
- Large lettuce leaves (e.g., butter lettuce, romaine)

Instructions:

- In a bowl, mix together tuna, mayonnaise, Dijon mustard, lemon juice, chopped celery, and chopped red onion (if using).
- Season with salt and pepper to taste.

- Spoon the tuna salad mixture onto large lettuce leaves.
- Wrap the lettuce leaves around the tuna salad to form lettuce wraps.
- Serve immediately and enjoy as a light and refreshing lunch option.

Health Benefits:

- Tuna is a lean source of protein and omega-3 fatty acids, promoting heart health and reducing inflammation.
- Celery provides fiber and antioxidants, supporting digestive health and immune function.
- Lettuce leaves offer a low-calorie, hydrating base for the wraps, adding vitamins and minerals to the meal.

Preparation Time: 10 minutes

6: Quinoa and Vegetable Stir-Fry

Ingredients:

- 1/2 cup quinoa, rinsed
- 1 cup water
- 1 tablespoon olive oil

- 1/2 cup sliced bell peppers (red, green, or yellow)
- 1/2 cup sliced zucchini
- 1/2 cup sliced carrots
- 1/4 cup sliced green onions
- 2 cloves garlic, minced
- 2 tablespoons low-sodium soy sauce (or tamari for gluten-free option)
- 1 tablespoon rice vinegar
- 1 teaspoon sesame oil (optional)
- Sesame seeds for garnish (optional)

Instructions:

- In a saucepan, combine quinoa and water. Bring to a boil, then reduce heat to low and simmer, covered, for 15 minutes or until quinoa is cooked and water is absorbed. Remove from heat and let it cool.
- Heat olive oil in a large skillet or wok over medium-high heat.
- Add sliced bell peppers, zucchini, carrots, green onions, and minced garlic to the skillet. Stir-fry for 5-7 minutes, or until vegetables are tender-crisp.

- Add cooked quinoa to the skillet and stir to combine with the vegetables.
- In a small bowl, whisk together soy sauce, rice vinegar, and sesame oil (if using). Pour the sauce over the quinoa and vegetable mixture.
- Cook for another 2-3 minutes, stirring occasionally, until heated through.
- Remove from heat and garnish with sesame seeds if desired.
- Serve immediately and enjoy as a flavorful and nutritious lunch option.

Health Benefits:

- Quinoa is a gluten-free whole grain rich in protein, fiber, and essential nutrients, providing sustained energy and promoting digestive health.
- Mixed vegetables offer vitamins, minerals, and antioxidants, supporting immune function and overall well-being.
- Soy sauce provides umami flavor and contains beneficial plant compounds, such as antioxidants and phytochemicals.

Preparation Time: 25 minutes

7: Quinoa and Chicken Soup

Ingredients:

- 1/2 cup quinoa, rinsed
- 4 cups low-sodium chicken broth
- 1 boneless, skinless chicken breast, cooked and shredded
- 1 cup mixed vegetables (e.g., carrots, celery, peas)
- 2 cloves garlic, minced
- 1 teaspoon dried thyme
- Salt and pepper to taste
- Fresh parsley for garnish (optional)

Instructions:

- In a large pot, bring the chicken broth to a boil over medium-high heat.
- Add quinoa, shredded chicken breast, mixed vegetables, minced garlic, and dried thyme to the pot.
- Reduce heat to low and simmer, covered, for 15-20 minutes, or until quinoa is cooked and vegetables are tender.

- Season with salt and pepper to taste.
- Ladle the soup into bowls and garnish with fresh parsley if desired.
- Serve hot and enjoy as a comforting and nourishing lunch option.

Health Benefits:

- Quinoa is a gluten-free whole grain rich in protein, fiber, and essential nutrients, providing sustained energy and promoting digestive health.
- Chicken broth provides hydration and electrolytes, supporting overall well-being and immune function.
- Mixed vegetables offer vitamins, minerals, and antioxidants, supporting digestive health and immune function.

Preparation Time: 30 minutes

8: Shrimp and Avocado Salad

Ingredients:

- 4 ounces cooked shrimp, peeled and deveined
- 1/2 avocado, diced

- 1 cup mixed salad greens (e.g., spinach, arugula, lettuce)
- 1/4 cup cherry tomatoes, halved
- 1/4 cup sliced cucumber
- 2 tablespoons chopped fresh cilantro
- 1 tablespoon olive oil
- 1 tablespoon lime juice
- Salt and pepper to taste

Instructions:

- In a large bowl, combine cooked shrimp, diced avocado, mixed salad greens, cherry tomatoes, sliced cucumber, and chopped cilantro.
- In a small bowl, whisk together olive oil, lime juice, salt, and pepper to make the dressing.
- Pour the dressing over the salad and toss gently to combine.
- Serve immediately and enjoy as a light and refreshing lunch option.

Health Benefits:

- Shrimp is a low-calorie source of protein and omega-3 fatty acids, promoting heart health and reducing inflammation.
- Avocado provides heart-healthy monounsaturated fats, fiber, and essential nutrients, promoting satiety and supporting digestive health.
- Mixed salad greens, cherry tomatoes, and cucumber offer vitamins, minerals, and antioxidants, supporting immune function and overall well-being.

Preparation Time: 15 minutes

9: Lentil and Vegetable Soup

Ingredients:

- 1 cup dried green lentils, rinsed
- 4 cups low-sodium vegetable broth
- 1 cup diced carrots
- 1 cup diced celery
- 1 cup diced potatoes
- 1/2 cup diced onion
- 2 cloves garlic, minced

- 1 teaspoon dried thyme
- Salt and pepper to taste
- Fresh parsley for garnish (optional)

Instructions:

- In a large pot, combine lentils, vegetable broth, carrots, celery, potatoes, onion, garlic, and thyme.
- Bring the mixture to a boil over medium-high heat, then reduce heat to low and simmer, covered, for 25-30 minutes, or until lentils and vegetables are tender.
- Season with salt and pepper to taste.
- Ladle the soup into bowls and garnish with fresh parsley if desired.
- Serve hot and enjoy as a comforting and nourishing lunch option.

Health Benefits:

- Lentils are a good source of plant-based protein, fiber, and essential nutrients, promoting digestive health and providing sustained energy.

- Vegetables such as carrots, celery, potatoes, and onions offer vitamins, minerals, and antioxidants, supporting immune function and overall well-being.
- Vegetable broth provides hydration and electrolytes, supporting hydration and aiding digestion.

Preparation Time: 40 minutes

10: Turkey and Vegetable Stir-Fry

Ingredients:

- 4 ounces cooked turkey breast, sliced
- 1 cup mixed vegetables (e.g., bell peppers, snap peas, broccoli florets)
- 2 cloves garlic, minced
- 1 tablespoon olive oil
- 2 tablespoons low-sodium soy sauce (or tamari for gluten-free option)
- 1 tablespoon rice vinegar
- 1 teaspoon sesame oil (optional)
- Sesame seeds for garnish (optional)
- Cooked rice or quinoa for serving

Instructions:

- Heat olive oil in a large skillet or wok over medium-high heat.
- Add sliced turkey breast, mixed vegetables, and minced garlic to the skillet. Stir-fry for 5-7 minutes, or until vegetables are tender-crisp.
- In a small bowl, whisk together soy sauce, rice vinegar, and sesame oil (if using). Pour the sauce over the turkey and vegetable mixture.
- Cook for another 2-3 minutes, stirring occasionally, until heated through.
- Remove from heat and garnish with sesame seeds if desired.
- Serve hot over cooked rice or quinoa and enjoy as a flavorful and nutritious lunch option.

Health Benefits:

- Turkey provides lean protein and essential amino acids necessary for muscle health and repair.
- Mixed vegetables offer vitamins, minerals, and antioxidants, supporting immune function and overall well-being.

- Soy sauce provides umami flavor and contains beneficial plant compounds, such as antioxidants and phytochemicals.

Preparation Time: 20 minutes

IBS Dinner Recipes for Seniors

1: Lemon Herb Baked Salmon with Quinoa and Steamed Vegetables

Ingredients:

- 2 salmon fillets
- 1 lemon, sliced
- 2 tablespoons olive oil
- 1 teaspoon dried thyme
- 1 teaspoon dried rosemary
- Salt and pepper to taste
- 1 cup quinoa
- 2 cups water or low-sodium chicken broth
- Mixed vegetables for steaming (e.g., carrots, zucchini, broccoli)

Instructions:

- Preheat the oven to 375°F (190°C).
- Place each salmon fillet on a piece of aluminum foil.
- Drizzle each salmon fillet with olive oil and season with dried thyme, dried rosemary, salt, and pepper. Top with lemon slices.
- Wrap the aluminum foil around the salmon fillets to create a packet.
- Place the salmon packets on a baking sheet and bake in the preheated oven for 15-20 minutes, or until the salmon is cooked through and flakes easily with a fork.
- While the salmon is baking, rinse the quinoa under cold water. In a saucepan, combine quinoa and water or low-sodium chicken broth. Bring to a boil, then reduce heat to low, cover, and simmer for 15 minutes, or until the quinoa is cooked and the liquid is absorbed.
- Steam mixed vegetables until tender, about 5-7 minutes.
- Serve the baked salmon with quinoa and steamed vegetables on the side.

Health Benefits:

- Salmon is rich in omega-3 fatty acids, which support heart health and reduce inflammation.
- Quinoa is a gluten-free whole grain that provides fiber, protein, and essential nutrients.
- Steamed vegetables are low in calories and high in fiber, vitamins, and minerals, supporting digestive health and overall well-being.

Preparation Time: 30 minutes

2: Turkey and Vegetable Stir-Fry with Brown Rice

Ingredients:

- 1 tablespoon olive oil
- 1 pound lean ground turkey
- 2 cups mixed vegetables (e.g., bell peppers, snap peas, carrots, broccoli)
- 2 cloves garlic, minced
- 1 tablespoon grated ginger
- 1/4 cup low-sodium soy sauce or tamari
- 2 cups cooked brown rice

Instructions:

- Heat olive oil in a large skillet or wok over medium heat.
- Add ground turkey to the skillet and cook until browned, breaking it apart with a spoon.
- Add mixed vegetables, minced garlic, and grated ginger to the skillet. Stir-fry for 5-7 minutes, or until the vegetables are tender-crisp.
- Pour low-sodium soy sauce or tamari over the turkey and vegetables. Stir to combine and cook for another 2-3 minutes.
- Serve the turkey and vegetable stir-fry over cooked brown rice.

Health Benefits:

- Lean ground turkey is a good source of protein and essential nutrients, supporting muscle health and overall well-being.
- Mixed vegetables provide vitamins, minerals, and antioxidants, promoting immune function and digestive health.

- Brown rice is a whole grain rich in fiber, which supports digestive regularity and heart health.

Preparation Time: 25 minutes

3: Baked Chicken Breast with Roasted Vegetables

Ingredients:

- 2 boneless, skinless chicken breasts
- 2 tablespoons olive oil
- 1 teaspoon dried Italian seasoning
- Salt and pepper to taste
- 2 cups mixed vegetables (e.g., bell peppers, onions, zucchini, cherry tomatoes)
- 1 tablespoon balsamic vinegar (optional)

Instructions:

- Preheat the oven to 400°F (200°C).
- Place the chicken breasts on a baking sheet lined with parchment paper or aluminum foil.
- Drizzle olive oil over the chicken breasts and season with dried Italian seasoning, salt, and pepper.

- Toss mixed vegetables with olive oil, salt, and pepper on a separate baking sheet.
- Place both baking sheets in the preheated oven. Bake chicken for 20-25 minutes, or until cooked through and no longer pink in the center. Roast vegetables for 15-20 minutes, or until tender and slightly caramelized.
- Optionally, drizzle roasted vegetables with balsamic vinegar before serving.
- Serve the baked chicken breasts with roasted vegetables on the side.

Health Benefits:

- Chicken breasts are a lean source of protein, essential for muscle health and overall well-being.
- Mixed vegetables are rich in fiber, vitamins, and minerals, supporting digestive health and immune function.
- Olive oil provides healthy fats and antioxidants, promoting heart health and reducing inflammation.

Preparation Time: 30 minutes

4: Quinoa and Black Bean Stuffed Bell Peppers

Ingredients:

- 4 large bell peppers (any color)
- 1 cup quinoa, rinsed
- 2 cups low-sodium vegetable broth
- 1 can (15 ounces) black beans, drained and rinsed
- 1 cup corn kernels (fresh, frozen, or canned)
- 1/2 cup diced tomatoes
- 1 teaspoon ground cumin
- 1/2 teaspoon chili powder
- Salt and pepper to taste
- 1/4 cup chopped fresh cilantro (optional)
- 1/4 cup shredded cheddar cheese (optional)

Instructions:

- Preheat the oven to 375°F (190°C).
- Cut the tops off the bell peppers and remove the seeds and membranes. Place the bell peppers upright in a baking dish.

- In a saucepan, combine quinoa and vegetable broth. Bring to a boil, then reduce heat to low, cover, and simmer for 15 minutes, or until the quinoa is cooked and the liquid is absorbed.
- In a large bowl, mix cooked quinoa, black beans, corn kernels, diced tomatoes, ground cumin, chili powder, salt, and pepper.
- Spoon the quinoa and black bean mixture into each bell pepper until filled.
- Cover the baking dish with aluminum foil and bake in the preheated oven for 25-30 minutes, or until the bell peppers are tender.
- Optionally, sprinkle stuffed bell peppers with chopped fresh cilantro and shredded cheddar cheese before serving.

Health Benefits:

- Quinoa is a gluten-free whole grain that provides fiber, protein, and essential nutrients, supporting digestive health and overall well-being.
- Black beans are rich in fiber and plant-based protein, promoting satiety and digestive regularity.

- Bell peppers are low in calories and high in vitamins, minerals, and antioxidants, supporting immune function and heart health.

Preparation Time: 45 minutes

5: Turkey and Vegetable Soup

Ingredients:

- 1 tablespoon olive oil
- 1 pound ground turkey
- 1 onion, diced
- 2 carrots, diced
- 2 celery stalks, diced
- 2 cloves garlic, minced
- 6 cups low-sodium chicken broth
- 1 can (14.5 ounces) diced tomatoes
- 1 teaspoon dried thyme
- 1 teaspoon dried oregano
- Salt and pepper to taste
- 2 cups chopped spinach or kale

Instructions:

- Heat olive oil in a large pot over medium heat.

- Add ground turkey to the pot and cook until browned, breaking it apart with a spoon.
- Add diced onion, carrots, celery, and minced garlic to the pot. Cook for 5-7 minutes, or until vegetables are tender.
- Pour low-sodium chicken broth and diced tomatoes into the pot. Stir in dried thyme, dried oregano, salt, and pepper.
- Bring the soup to a boil, then reduce heat to low and simmer for 20-25 minutes, allowing flavors to meld.
- Stir in chopped spinach or kale and cook for an additional 5 minutes, or until greens are wilted.
- Taste and adjust seasoning if necessary.
- Serve hot and enjoy as a comforting and nourishing dinner option.

Health Benefits:

- Ground turkey is a lean source of protein and essential nutrients, supporting muscle health and overall well-being.

- Vegetables provide vitamins, minerals, and antioxidants, promoting immune function and digestive health.
- Homemade soup is hydrating and easy to digest, making it ideal for seniors with IBS.

Preparation Time: 40 minutes

6: Baked Cod with Lemon and Herbs

Ingredients:

- 4 cod fillets
- 2 tablespoons olive oil
- 1 lemon, thinly sliced
- 2 cloves garlic, minced
- 1 teaspoon dried thyme
- 1 teaspoon dried parsley
- Salt and pepper to taste

Instructions:

- Preheat the oven to 375°F (190°C).
- Place the cod fillets on a baking sheet lined with parchment paper or aluminum foil.

- Drizzle olive oil over the cod fillets and season with minced garlic, dried thyme, dried parsley, salt, and pepper.
- Top each cod fillet with lemon slices.
- Bake in the preheated oven for 15-20 minutes, or until the cod is cooked through and flakes easily with a fork.
- Serve hot and enjoy with your choice of side dishes, such as steamed vegetables or quinoa.

Health Benefits:

- Cod is a lean source of protein and omega-3 fatty acids, which support heart health and reduce inflammation.
- Olive oil provides healthy fats and antioxidants, promoting heart health and reducing inflammation.
- Lemon and herbs add flavor without added sodium or calories, enhancing the taste of the dish.

Preparation Time: 20 minutes

7: Grilled Chicken and Vegetable Skewers

Ingredients:

- 2 boneless, skinless chicken breasts, cut into cubes
- 1 zucchini, sliced
- 1 bell pepper, cut into chunks
- 1 red onion, cut into chunks
- 8 cherry tomatoes
- 2 tablespoons olive oil
- 2 cloves garlic, minced
- 1 teaspoon dried oregano
- 1 teaspoon dried thyme
- Salt and pepper to taste
- Wooden skewers, soaked in water for 30 minutes

Instructions:

- In a bowl, combine chicken cubes, sliced zucchini, bell pepper chunks, red onion chunks, and cherry tomatoes.
- In a small bowl, whisk together olive oil, minced garlic, dried oregano, dried thyme, salt, and pepper to make the marinade.

- Pour the marinade over the chicken and vegetables, tossing to coat evenly. Marinate in the refrigerator for at least 30 minutes.
- Preheat the grill to medium-high heat.
- Thread the marinated chicken and vegetables onto the soaked wooden skewers, alternating between ingredients.
- Place the skewers on the preheated grill and cook for 10-12 minutes, turning occasionally, or until the chicken is cooked through and the vegetables are tender and slightly charred.
- Serve the grilled chicken and vegetable skewers hot with your choice of side dishes, such as quinoa or brown rice.

Health Benefits:

- Chicken breast is a lean source of protein, essential for muscle health and overall well-being.
- Vegetables provide fiber, vitamins, and minerals, supporting digestive health and immune function.
- Grilling reduces the need for added fats, making this dish heart-healthy and suitable for seniors with IBS.

Preparation Time: 40 minutes (including marinating time)

8: Turkey and Quinoa Stuffed Bell Peppers

Ingredients:

- 4 large bell peppers (any color)
- 1 tablespoon olive oil
- 1 onion, diced
- 2 cloves garlic, minced
- 1 pound lean ground turkey
- 1 cup cooked quinoa
- 1 can (14.5 ounces) diced tomatoes
- 1 teaspoon dried oregano
- 1 teaspoon dried basil
- Salt and pepper to taste
- 1/4 cup grated Parmesan cheese (optional)

Instructions:

- Preheat the oven to 375°F (190°C).
- Cut the tops off the bell peppers and remove the seeds and membranes. Place the bell peppers upright in a baking dish.

- In a skillet, heat olive oil over medium heat. Add diced onion and minced garlic, cooking until softened.
- Add ground turkey to the skillet and cook until browned, breaking it apart with a spoon.
- Stir in cooked quinoa, diced tomatoes, dried oregano, dried basil, salt, and pepper. Cook for 5 minutes, allowing flavors to meld.
- Spoon the turkey and quinoa mixture into each bell pepper until filled.
- Cover the baking dish with aluminum foil and bake in the preheated oven for 25-30 minutes, or until the bell peppers are tender.
- Optionally, sprinkle stuffed bell peppers with grated Parmesan cheese before serving.

Health Benefits:

- Lean ground turkey provides protein, essential for muscle health and overall well-being.
- Quinoa is a gluten-free whole grain that offers fiber and essential nutrients, supporting digestive health and immune function.

- Bell peppers are low in calories and high in vitamins, minerals, and antioxidants, promoting heart health and digestive health.

Preparation Time: 45 minutes

9: Salmon and Vegetable Foil Packets

Ingredients:

- 2 salmon fillets
- 1 zucchini, sliced
- 1 yellow squash, sliced
- 1 bell pepper, sliced
- 1/2 red onion, sliced
- 2 tablespoons olive oil
- 2 cloves garlic, minced
- 1 teaspoon dried dill
- Salt and pepper to taste
- Lemon wedges for serving

Instructions:

- Preheat the oven to 400°F (200°C).
- Place each salmon fillet in the center of a large piece of aluminum foil.

- In a bowl, toss sliced zucchini, yellow squash, bell pepper, and red onion with olive oil, minced garlic, dried dill, salt, and pepper.
- Divide the vegetable mixture evenly between the two foil packets, placing them on top of the salmon fillets.
- Fold the edges of the foil to seal the packets, leaving some room for steam to circulate.
- Place the foil packets on a baking sheet and bake in the preheated oven for 15-20 minutes, or until the salmon is cooked through and flakes easily with a fork.
- Carefully open the foil packets and transfer the contents to plates.
- Serve hot with lemon wedges for squeezing over the salmon and vegetables.

Health Benefits:

Salmon is a rich source of omega-3 fatty acids, which support heart health and reduce inflammation.

Zucchini, yellow squash, bell pepper, and red onion provide fiber, vitamins, and minerals, promoting digestive health and immune function.

This dish is baked in foil packets, which helps to retain moisture and flavor without added fats, making it gentle on the digestive system.

Preparation Time: 25 minutes

10: Turkey and Vegetable Quinoa Bowl

Ingredients:

- 1 cup quinoa, rinsed
- 2 cups low-sodium chicken broth
- 1 tablespoon olive oil
- 1 pound lean ground turkey
- 1 teaspoon ground cumin
- 1 teaspoon paprika
- Salt and pepper to taste
- 1 zucchini, diced
- 1 yellow squash, diced
- 1 bell pepper, diced
- 1/2 cup cherry tomatoes, halved

- 1/4 cup chopped fresh parsley

Instructions:

- In a saucepan, combine quinoa and low-sodium chicken broth. Bring to a boil, then reduce heat to low, cover, and simmer for 15 minutes, or until the quinoa is cooked and the liquid is absorbed.
- Heat olive oil in a large skillet over medium heat. Add ground turkey and cook until browned, breaking it apart with a spoon.
- Stir in ground cumin, paprika, salt, and pepper. Add diced zucchini, yellow squash, and bell pepper to the skillet. Cook for 5-7 minutes, or until vegetables are tender.
- Add cooked quinoa and cherry tomatoes to the skillet, stirring to combine. Cook for another 2-3 minutes to heat through.
- Remove from heat and stir in chopped fresh parsley.
- Serve hot in bowls and enjoy as a balanced and satisfying dinner.

Health Benefits:

- Quinoa is a gluten-free whole grain that provides fiber, protein, and essential nutrients, supporting digestive health and overall well-being.
- Lean ground turkey offers protein and essential nutrients, promoting muscle health and satiety.
- Zucchini, yellow squash, bell pepper, cherry tomatoes, and parsley provide vitamins, minerals, and antioxidants, supporting immune function and heart health.

Preparation Time: 30 minutes

IBS Snacks Recipes for Seniors

1: Rice Cake with Avocado and Tomato

Ingredients:

- 1 rice cake (gluten-free if necessary)
- 1/4 ripe avocado, mashed
- 1 small tomato, thinly sliced
- Pinch of sea salt
- Pinch of black pepper

- Optional: fresh basil leaves or drizzle of balsamic glaze

Instructions:

- Spread mashed avocado evenly over the rice cake.
- Top with thinly sliced tomato.
- Season with a pinch of sea salt and black pepper.
- Optional: Garnish with fresh basil leaves or drizzle with balsamic glaze for extra flavor.
- Serve immediately and enjoy as a satisfying and nutritious snack.

Health Benefits:

- Avocado is a good source of healthy fats, fiber, and vitamins, supporting heart health and digestive function.
- Tomatoes provide antioxidants, vitamins, and minerals, promoting immune function and overall well-being.
- Rice cakes are a gluten-free, low-FODMAP option for individuals with IBS, offering a light and crunchy base for the snack.

Preparation Time: 5 minutes

2: Greek Yogurt with Berries and Almonds

Ingredients:

- 1/2 cup lactose-free Greek yogurt or coconut yogurt
- 1/4 cup mixed berries (e.g., strawberries, blueberries, raspberries)
- 1 tablespoon slivered almonds or chopped walnuts
- Drizzle of honey or maple syrup (optional)

Instructions:

- Spoon Greek yogurt into a small bowl or serving dish.
- Top with mixed berries and slivered almonds or chopped walnuts.
- Drizzle with honey or maple syrup if desired for added sweetness.
- Serve immediately and enjoy as a delicious and satisfying snack.

Health Benefits:

- Greek yogurt is rich in protein and probiotics, supporting digestive health and immune function.

- Berries are packed with antioxidants, vitamins, and fiber, promoting heart health and overall well-being.
- Almonds and walnuts provide healthy fats, protein, and essential nutrients, supporting brain health and satiety.

Preparation Time: 5 minutes

3: Carrot Sticks with Hummus

Ingredients:

- 2 medium carrots, peeled and cut into sticks
- 1/4 cup low-FODMAP hummus (store-bought or homemade)
- Optional: paprika, cumin, or fresh herbs for garnish

Instructions:

- Wash, peel, and cut carrots into sticks.
- Serve carrot sticks with low-FODMAP hummus for dipping.
- Optional: Garnish hummus with a sprinkle of paprika, cumin, or fresh herbs for extra flavor.
- Enjoy immediately as a crunchy and satisfying snack.

Health Benefits:

- Carrots are rich in beta-carotene, vitamins, and fiber, promoting eye health and digestive regularity.
- Hummus provides plant-based protein, fiber, and healthy fats, supporting satiety and heart health.
- This snack is low in FODMAPs, making it suitable for individuals with IBS and sensitive digestive systems.

Preparation Time: 5 minutes

4: Rice Cake with Almond Butter and Banana

Ingredients:

- 1 rice cake (gluten-free if necessary)
- 1 tablespoon natural almond butter
- 1/2 ripe banana, thinly sliced
- Optional: sprinkle of cinnamon or drizzle of honey

Instructions:

- Spread almond butter evenly over the rice cake.
- Top with thinly sliced banana.

- Optional: Sprinkle with cinnamon or drizzle with honey for added sweetness.
- Serve immediately and enjoy as a quick and nutritious snack.

Health Benefits:

- Almond butter provides healthy fats, protein, and essential nutrients, supporting heart health and energy levels.
- Bananas are a good source of potassium, fiber, and vitamins, promoting digestive health and muscle function.
- Rice cakes are a low-FODMAP, gluten-free option for individuals with IBS, offering a light and crunchy base for the snack.

Preparation Time: 5 minutes

5: Quinoa Salad with Cucumber and Feta

Ingredients:

- 1/2 cup cooked quinoa, cooled
- 1/4 cucumber, diced
- 2 tablespoons crumbled feta cheese

- 1 tablespoon chopped fresh parsley
- 1 tablespoon lemon juice
- 1 tablespoon extra virgin olive oil
- Salt and pepper to taste

Instructions:

- In a bowl, combine cooked quinoa, diced cucumber, crumbled feta cheese, and chopped fresh parsley.
- Drizzle with lemon juice and extra virgin olive oil.
- Season with salt and pepper to taste.
- Toss gently to combine all ingredients.
- Serve immediately or refrigerate until ready to eat.
- Enjoy chilled as a refreshing and nutritious snack.

Health Benefits:

- Quinoa is a gluten-free whole grain that provides protein, fiber, and essential nutrients, supporting digestive health and overall well-being.
- Cucumber is hydrating and low in calories, while also providing vitamins and minerals that support hydration and digestive health.

- Feta cheese adds flavor and calcium, promoting bone health and muscle function.

Preparation Time: 15 minutes

6: Rice Crackers with Tuna Salad

Ingredients:

- 4 rice crackers (gluten-free if necessary)
- 1/2 cup canned tuna, drained
- 2 tablespoons plain Greek yogurt
- 1 tablespoon diced celery
- 1 tablespoon diced red bell pepper
- 1 tablespoon chopped fresh parsley
- Salt and pepper to taste

Instructions:

- In a bowl, mix together drained tuna, plain Greek yogurt, diced celery, diced red bell pepper, and chopped fresh parsley.
- Season with salt and pepper to taste.
- Spoon tuna salad onto rice crackers, dividing evenly among them.

- Serve immediately and enjoy as a protein-rich and satisfying snack.

Health Benefits:

- Tuna is a lean source of protein and omega-3 fatty acids, which support heart health and muscle function.
- Greek yogurt adds creaminess and probiotics, supporting digestive health and immune function.
- Rice crackers are a gluten-free option for individuals with IBS, providing a crunchy base for the snack.

Preparation Time: 10 minutes

7: Baked Sweet Potato Chips

Ingredients:

- 1 medium sweet potato, thinly sliced
- 1 tablespoon olive oil
- 1/2 teaspoon smoked paprika
- 1/4 teaspoon garlic powder
- Salt to taste

Instructions:

- Preheat the oven to 375°F (190°C) and line a baking sheet with parchment paper.
- In a bowl, toss the thinly sliced sweet potato with olive oil, smoked paprika, garlic powder, and salt until evenly coated.
- Arrange the sweet potato slices in a single layer on the prepared baking sheet.
- Bake for 15-20 minutes, flipping halfway through, or until the sweet potato chips are crispy and golden brown.
- Remove from the oven and let cool slightly before serving.
- Enjoy the baked sweet potato chips as a crunchy and nutritious snack.

Health Benefits:

- Sweet potatoes are rich in vitamins, minerals, and fiber, supporting digestive health and immune function.
- Olive oil provides healthy fats and antioxidants, promoting heart health and reducing inflammation.

- Baking instead of frying reduces the fat content and makes this snack more suitable for seniors with IBS.

Preparation Time: 25 minutes

8: Cottage Cheese with Pineapple

Ingredients:

- 1/2 cup lactose-free cottage cheese or Greek yogurt
- 1/2 cup fresh pineapple chunks
- Optional: drizzle of honey or sprinkle of cinnamon

Instructions:

- Spoon lactose-free cottage cheese or Greek yogurt into a small bowl or serving dish.
- Top with fresh pineapple chunks.
- Optional: Drizzle with honey or sprinkle with cinnamon for added sweetness and flavor.
- Serve immediately and enjoy as a protein-rich and satisfying snack.

Health Benefits:

- Cottage cheese or Greek yogurt provides protein and probiotics, supporting digestive health and muscle function.
- Pineapple is rich in vitamin C, bromelain, and fiber, promoting immune function and digestive regularity.
- This snack is low in FODMAPs and easy to digest, making it suitable for individuals with IBS.

Preparation Time: 5 minutes

9: Almond Butter and Banana Roll-Ups

Ingredients:

- 1 whole grain tortilla (gluten-free if necessary)
- 2 tablespoons natural almond butter
- 1/2 ripe banana, peeled
- Optional: sprinkle of cinnamon or drizzle of honey

Instructions:

- Lay the whole grain tortilla flat on a clean surface.
- Spread almond butter evenly over the tortilla.
- Place the banana in the center of the tortilla.

- Optional: Sprinkle with cinnamon or drizzle with honey for added flavor.
- Roll up the tortilla tightly, enclosing the banana.
- Slice the roll-up into bite-sized pieces.
- Serve immediately and enjoy as a delicious and satisfying snack.

Health Benefits:

- Almond butter provides healthy fats, protein, and essential nutrients, supporting heart health and energy levels.
- Bananas are a good source of potassium, fiber, and vitamins, promoting digestive health and muscle function.
- Whole grain tortillas offer fiber and complex carbohydrates, providing sustained energy and digestive regularity.

Preparation Time: 5 minutes

10: Veggie Sticks with Yogurt Dip

Ingredients:

- Assorted vegetable sticks (e.g., carrot, cucumber, bell pepper)
- 1/2 cup lactose-free Greek yogurt or coconut yogurt
- 1 tablespoon chopped fresh dill or parsley
- 1/2 teaspoon lemon juice
- Salt and pepper to taste

Instructions:

- Wash and prepare assorted vegetable sticks, cutting them into manageable sizes for dipping.
- In a bowl, mix together lactose-free Greek yogurt or coconut yogurt, chopped fresh dill or parsley, lemon juice, salt, and pepper.
- Transfer the yogurt dip to a serving bowl.
- Arrange the vegetable sticks on a platter around the yogurt dip.
- Serve immediately and enjoy as a crunchy and nutritious snack.

Health Benefits:

- Assorted vegetable sticks provide vitamins, minerals, and fiber, supporting digestive health and immune function.
- Lactose-free Greek yogurt or coconut yogurt offers probiotics and protein, promoting gut health and satiety.
- This snack is low in FODMAPs and easy to digest, making it suitable for individuals with IBS.

Preparation Time: 10 minutes

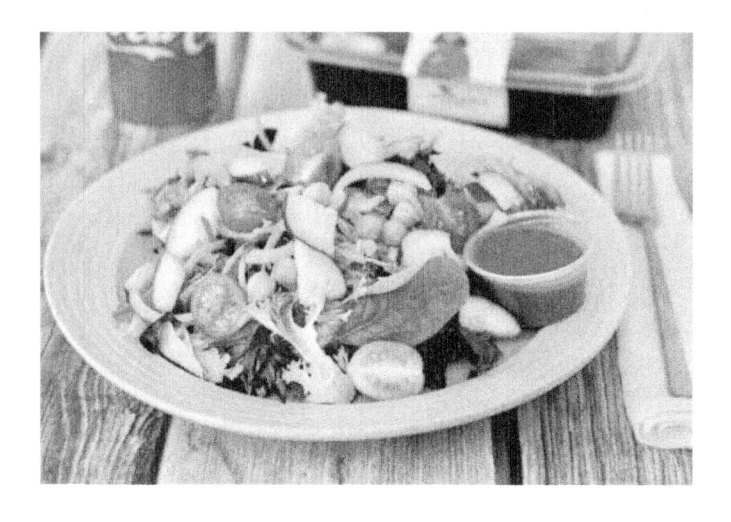

CONCLUSION

The IBS Recipes Cookbook for Seniors offers a diverse array of delicious, nutritious, and easy-to-make recipes tailored specifically for individuals managing Irritable Bowel Syndrome (IBS) in their golden years.

From hearty breakfast options to satisfying snacks, each recipe is thoughtfully crafted to accommodate the unique dietary needs and sensitivities of seniors with IBS.

By incorporating low-FODMAP ingredients, gentle cooking techniques, and digestive-friendly foods, this cookbook provides seniors with practical solutions to alleviate symptoms and improve overall well-being.

Whether enjoying a comforting bowl of oatmeal, a refreshing smoothie, or a crunchy vegetable snack, seniors can indulge in flavorful dishes without compromising their digestive health.

Beyond the recipes themselves, this cookbook serves as a valuable resource, offering insightful tips, nutritional guidance, and practical advice for managing IBS symptoms effectively.

With an emphasis on whole, nutrient-rich ingredients and mindful eating habits, seniors can cultivate a positive relationship with food and nourish their bodies in a way that promotes digestive comfort and vitality.

In embracing the recipes and principles outlined in this cookbook, seniors can embark on a journey towards improved digestive health, enhanced quality of life, and culinary enjoyment.

With each meal prepared with care and intention, seniors can savor the pleasures of good food while supporting their digestive wellness for years to come.

Printed in Great Britain
by Amazon